Rescuing Rover

A First Aid and Disaster Guide for Dog Owners

Sebastian E. Heath and Andrea O'Shea

Rescuing Rover

A First Aid and Disaster Guide for Dog Owners

Sebastian E. Heath and Andrea O'Shea

Purdue University Press / West Lafayette, Indiana

For all procedures indicated and recommendations made in this book, you should work closely under the supervision of a veterinarian.

Neither the authors of the book nor Purdue University Press make representation or warranty whatsoever regarding (i) the effectiveness of any product mentioned herein; or (ii) the effectiveness of a particular method, technique or process addressed herein, under extreme conditions occasioned by any disaster. The ideas expressed in this book are merely set forth as suggestive to the reader of the types of issues with which he or she should be concerned in maintaining the safety of his or her dog and are not intended as an all-inclusive list for preparedness in the event of any disaster.

03   02   01   00   99   5   4   3   2   1

The paper used in this book meets the minimum requirements of American National Standard for Information Sciences—Permanence of Paper for Printed Library Materials, ANSI Z39.48-1992.

Printed in the United States of America

Medical procedures illustrated by Andrea O'Shea

Cover illustration and interior design by David Black

Library of Congress Cataloging-in-Publication Data

Heath, Sebastian E., 1955–
      Rescuing rover : a first aid and disaster guide for dog owners / Sebastian E. Heath and Andrea O'Shea.
            p.   cm.
      ISBN 1-55753-102-1 (pbk. : alk. paper)
      1. Dogs—Wounds and injuries—Treatment. 2. Dogs—Diseases—Treatment. 3. First aid for animals. 4. Veterinary emergencies.
      I. O'Shea, Andrea, 1952– . II. Title.
      SF991.H435 1998
      636.7'08960252—dc21   98-53503
                                                                              CIP

Contents

Contents (cont'd)

Introduction

This book originated from the needs of canine search and rescue teams, who work under conditions where veterinary services may not be available. If a search dog is injured in the field, it may have to be treated by a physician or emergency medical technician. Under these conditions, handlers and emergency physicians need a practical guide to provide optimum care for the dog until it can be transported to a veterinarian. As we looked into the available materials on first aid for dogs, we also found that there is an even broader need for practical first-aid materials among dog owners and handlers. So we set out to identify common, serious first-aid issues that dogs and their handlers are likely to encounter and compiled some practical solutions.

This book should not replace the extensive knowledge and expertise of veterinary specialists. It is intended to guide owners and handlers to prepare an injured dog so that it can be safely transported to a veterinarian without further harm to the dog or handler. It can also be used as a practical learning guide for veterinary medical and technician students and as a teaching tool for veterinary specialists teaching first aid. Some of the advanced procedures should be reserved for qualified veterinary health professionals. We have included these procedures so that owners and handlers can be of optimum help to veterinary care providers under emergency conditions.

Owners and handlers can prepare for emergencies by practicing the restraint and muzzling procedures on their dogs. If a dog is familiar with these procedures, it will be less stressed when it needs help most, and further injury to the dog and persons will be less likely. We strongly recommend that all dogs pay regular visits to a veterinarian, attend obedience classes, and be frequently socialized with people of all ages and other dogs. Practicing bandaging is a fun and effective way to socialize a dog, learn the technique, and familiarize the dog with what to expect in an emergency.

We have limited ourselves to selected common emergencies and maintain that the best intervention is to prevent emergencies from occurring in the first place. However, some disasters will unfortunately always occur, and the best that one can do to reduce their impact is to be prepared. We hope that this book improves the quality of care for dogs and heightens people's awareness for increased safety in our interactions with dogs.

We would like to thank Jean Hooks and Karen Cornell for their help in preparing this book.

Rescuing Rover

Restraint Techniques

Principle

This section shows dog owners and handlers the appropriate methods for restraining a dog so that a qualified veterinary medical professional can safely attend to it.

Procedure

Lateral Restraint (A)

1. Command the dog to lie down.

2. Kneel with knees against the dog's back.

3. Place left forearm on the dog's neck; hold the dog's lower (left) front limb with left hand.

4. Place right arm across the dog's flank; hold the dog's lower (left) hind limb with right hand.

5. Shift your weight over the dog's body.

Seated Restraint (B)

1. Command the dog to sit.

2. Kneel behind the dog.

3. With your left arm, reach under the dog's neck and hold the dog's head in a locked position.

4. With your right arm, grasp the dog's right elbow and extend this joint.

4

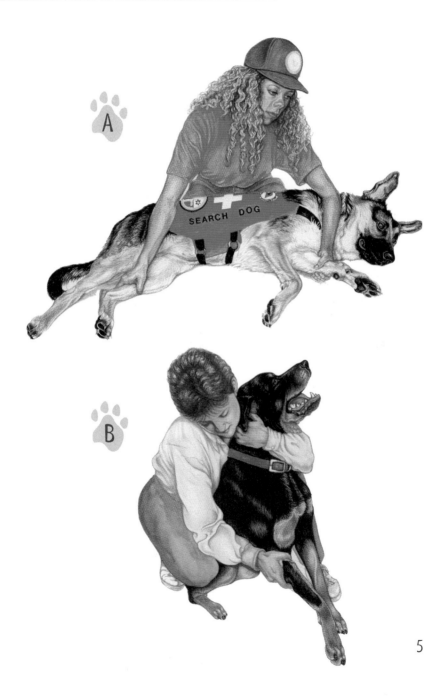

A

B

Muzzling a Dog

Principle

When a dog is frightened or in pain, a muzzle is needed to protect people treating the dog from being bitten. This section shows owners and handlers the appropriate method for muzzling a dog when a fitted muzzle is unavailable. A fitted muzzle obviously is best.

Procedure

1. Place a 2-inch-wide gauze tape approximately 4 feet long under the dog's jaw.

2. Circle the gauze around the dog's muzzle. Tie a half-knot above the nose and tighten.

3. Bring the loose ends of the gauze back under the jaw. Tie another half-knot and tighten.

4. Bring the loose ends of the gauze under and behind the ears and tie in a firm bow at the back of the neck.

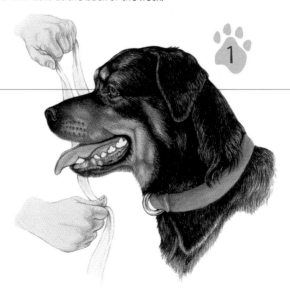

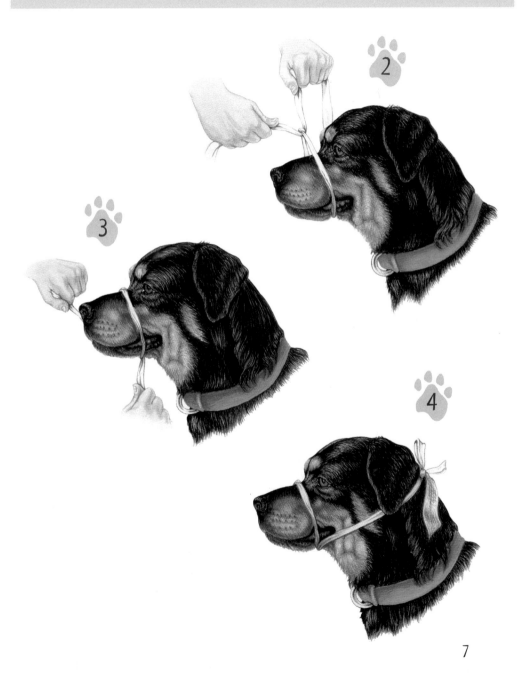

Examining and Treating the Eye

Principle

Common irritants to the eye are dust, pollen, and foreign bodies. A common sign of irritation is excessive squinting. Sometimes dogs will also scratch at an irritated eye, which can quickly make it worse. This section shows dog owners and handlers how to restrain a dog for examination and treatment of an irritated or injured eye and demonstrates this procedure for nonveterinary medically trained personnel. Nonqualified persons should never perform this procedure. An irritated or injured eye should always be thoroughly examined by a veterinarian.

A dog's eye should be approached with instruments or drops from above and behind the frontal plane.

Procedure

Restrain the dog in a sitting position. (See p. 5.)

1. Hold the dog's head with one hand around the jaw, gently pulling down the lower eyelid. With the other hand pull up the upper lid. Then a medical professional can administer saline or anesthetic drops or flushes to the affected eye from above.

2. Once the eye is anesthetized, a medical professional should examine under the third eyelid using a nontraumatic thumb forceps. His/her hand should rest on the dog's cheek under the affected eye, gently grasp the third eyelid with the forceps, and pull it out to expose the entire underside of the lid.

3. If a foreign body is found, a saline solution should be used to flush it out. If this does not remove the irritant, a cotton-tipped swab can be used to gently dislodge it. If it cannot be dislodged, bandage the entire eye shut and immediately seek veterinary advice.

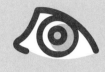

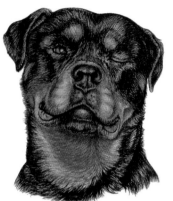

dog with injured eye

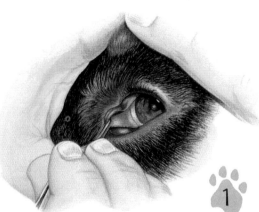

1

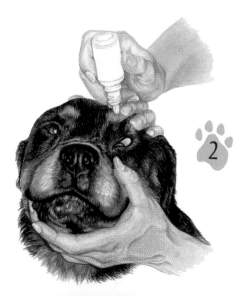

2

9

Bandaging Upright Ears

Principle

Bandaging an injured ear prevents further damage, which can result from the dog scratching the affected ear. Bandaging also prevents blood spattering when the dog shakes its head. Always have injuries examined by a veterinarian.

Procedure

1. Fill the inside of the ear with a ball of cotton wool. If possible, cover the wound with a gauze pad.

2. Fold the ear forward onto the dog's head. Cover the back of the ear with a gauze pad.

3–5. Gently wrap a gauze bandage over the ear and gauze pad.

6. The wrap should cover the affected ear from behind and in front. Leave plenty of room for the uninjured ear to move. Secure the gauze wrap with tape.

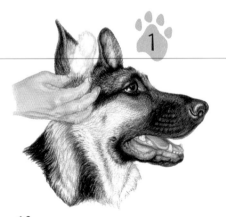
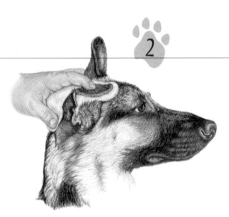

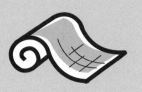

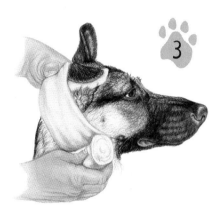

3

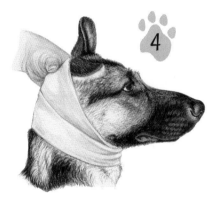

4

5

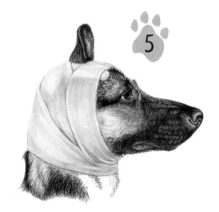

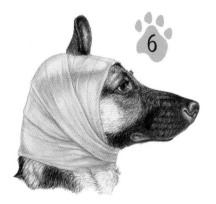

6

Bandaging Floppy Ears

Principle

Bandaging an injured ear prevents further injury, which can result from the dog scratching the affected ear, and prevents blood spattering when the dog shakes its head. In this example the dog has a semifloppy right ear. Always have injuries examined by a veterinarian.

Procedure

1. Place a gauze pad behind the ear and fold the ear over the gauze onto the dog's head.

2. Cover the inside of the ear (now exposed to the outside) with another gauze pad.

3-4. Gently wrap a gauze bandage over the ear and the gauze pads. Leave plenty of room for the other, uninjured ear to move freely.

5. Secure the gauze wrap with tape.

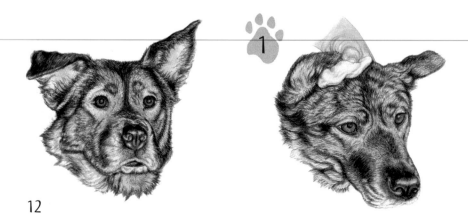

1

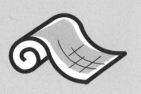

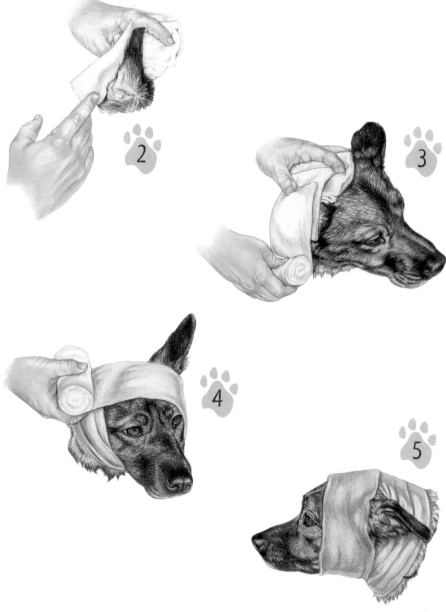

Foot Injuries and Bandaging

Procedure

A. Cut Foot Pad

- Restrain the dog in a lateral position.

- Apply pressure until bleeding stops (this injury commonly bleeds a lot).

- Flush the wound with a saline solution until clean, then flush the wound with an antiseptic solution.

- Bandage as described below.

B. Broken or Fractured Toenail

- This injury can be very painful, so muzzle the dog before any examination or treatment.

- Restrain the dog in a lateral position.

- Using forceps, firmly grasp the toenail and quickly twist off the nail in the direction in which it is deviated.

- Bandage as described below.

Bandaging

1. Dry the foot and put strips of cotton between the toes.

2. Cover the affected pad or toenail with a nonstick dressing.

3-4. Cover the walking surface of the foot with gauze squares.

(continued on page 16)

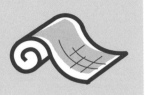

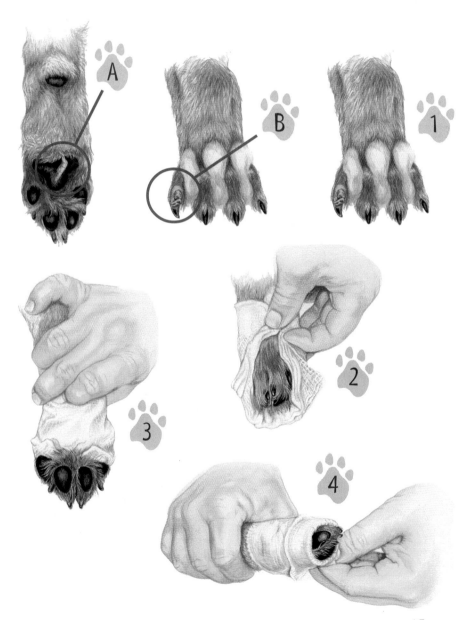

Bandaging (continued from page 14)

5. Wrap the foot with cotton. The cotton wrap should leave the two center toes exposed and extend to 1 inch above where the top of the adhesive bandage will be.

6. Wrap the cotton-covered foot with stretch gauze using gentle, even pressure.

7. Be sure the bandage is only so tight that your finger can fit between the middle toes of the dog. This will allow normal blood flow.

8. Complete the bandage with a final layer of adhesive elastic wrap. To keep the bandage from slipping, incorporate some hair into the tape at top of bandage.

9. The exposed cotton wool can be folded back onto the bandage and secured with 2-inch adhesive tape.

Always have injuries examined by a veterinarian.

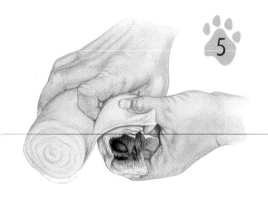

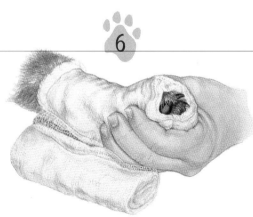

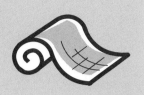

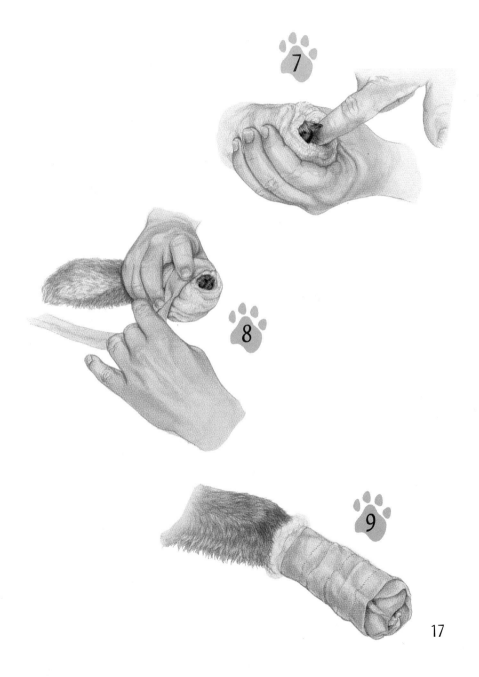

Bandaging the Lower Leg

Principle

A very thick bandage can be used as a splint if a dog breaks its leg or dislocates a joint below the stifle (knee) or elbow. This is only a temporary splint; consult a veterinarian as soon as possible. The following example shows the procedure for the right hind leg.

Procedure

1. Stick two 1-inch-wide strips of adhesive tape to either side of the dog's leg, from the toe to the hock. Leave about 1 foot of tape free beyond the toe.

2–3. Wrap the leg several inches thick with cotton. The inside surface should have as few folds as possible.

4. Tightly wrap the cotton with cling gauze.

5. Stick the free ends of the adhesive tape to either side of the cling gauze.

6. Complete the bandage by firmly wrapping elastic adhesive tape around the outside. The final bandage should be about as thick as the dog's waist.

7. Leave the tips of the toes exposed. Leave the top of the cotton bandage exposed, or fold it down and cover it with tape.

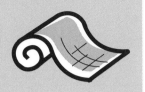

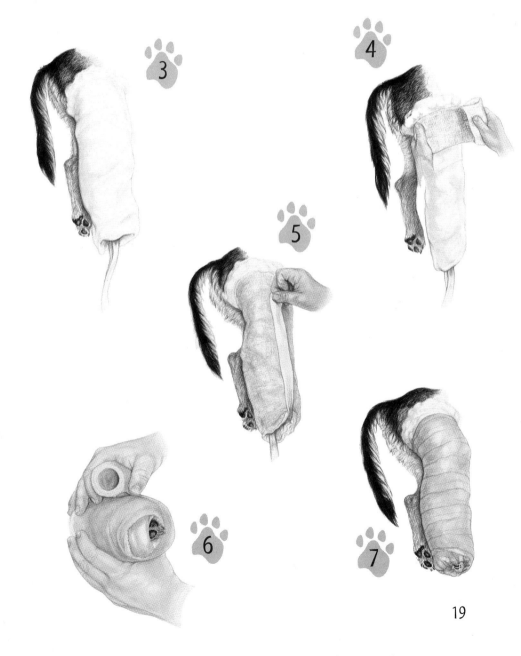

Bandaging the Tail

Principle

Bandaging an injured tail prevents further injury and keeps blood from spattering when the dog wags its tail. Injuries high on the tail do not require the entire tail to be bandaged. A tail bandage should be as light as possible and be applied with enough pressure to ensure that normal circulation of blood continues. As in the case of all injuries, clean the injured site and prepare it by trimming the hair in the vicinity of the injury.

Procedure

1. Cover the injury with an absorbent gauze pad.

2. Wrap the injured part of the tail with 1 or 2 layers of cotton gauze.

3. Wrap the cotton with cling gauze.

4. Make sure that the hair is folded away from the bandage.

5. Complete the bandage with a layer of adhesive elastic tape.

6. Incorporate some of the hair of the tail under the final layer of the adhesive tape to act as an anchor for the bandage.

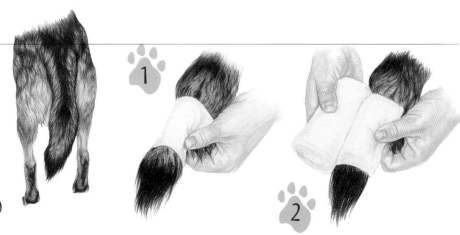

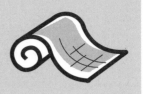

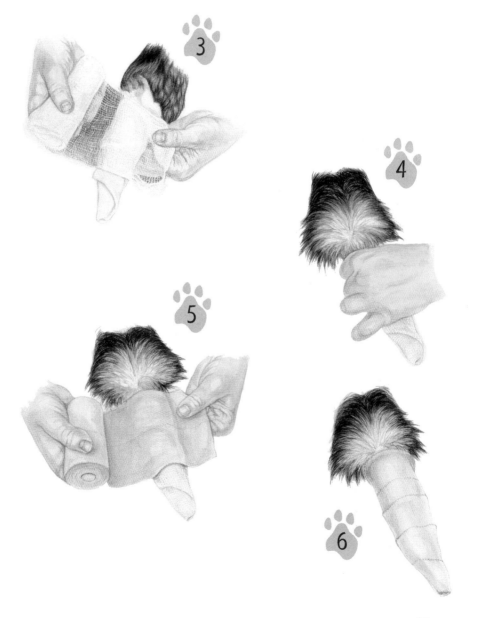

Medical Emergencies

Seek professional veterinary advice for any medical problem that your dog may have. Under certain conditions emergencies will occur, but much can be done to prevent them from getting worse. Make sure that your dog is current on vaccinations and parasite-control medication. Work or exercise your dog only if he or she is physically fit. A sound nutritional and exercise program is paramount to good health. Working dogs should always be maintained on their staple diet when away from home. Changes in a dog's diet, including feeding unfamiliar tidbits or treats, can lead to diarrhea and other conditions.

The scope of this book does not allow a comprehensive list of medical emergencies, so we are limiting ourselves to cursory descriptions of some common conditions in dogs. We specifically refrain from advising treatments to discourage people from treating their animals without consulting a veterinarian.

You can help your dog by knowing its normal resting heart rate and temperature. You should also know how to measure these and your dog's pulse and capillary refill time. Written copies of your dog's medical history, including vaccination status, should accompany him/her at all times. Consult your regular veterinarian about these procedures and he or she will be able to provide this information. A veterinarian or veterinary technician can also show you how to take your dog's pulse and temperature, and to examine its mucous membranes.

Shock

Shock results from circulatory failure. Dogs in shock are weak and lethargic, or may collapse. Their heart rate is persistently elevated, pulse may be weak, the mucous membranes are pale, and the capillary refill time is slow. Shock is often

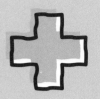

associated with dehydration, which may be the result of excessive fluid loss or inadequate fluid intake. Excessive fluid losses occur during work or extreme exercise and can be exacerbated by medical conditions such as diarrhea and kidney disease. Other factors that can lead to shock are ill health, overworking, work in hot climates (hyperthermia) or excessively cold climates (hypothermia), exhaustion, heart failure, and exposure to toxins. If you think your dog is in shock, do NOT exercise him or her further. Seek veterinary advice immediately.

Diarrhea

There are many causes of diarrhea, including excitement or changes in food and water. Diarrhea can be a life-threatening condition, and the extensive fluid loss can lead to shock and death. The cause of the diarrhea should always be established by a veterinarian so that appropriate preventive and therapeutic treatments can be made.

Insect and Snake Bites

Insect and snake bites occur relatively often in working dogs and can occur when exercising your dog in remote areas. For some snake venoms there are specific antidotes, but they are effective only if the snake has been correctly identified.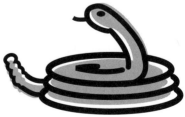
Therefore, always try to get a good description of the snake without endangering yourself in the process. For symptomatic treatment for insect and snake bites, cover the bite site with ice packs until veterinary advice can be obtained. Ice packs cool the site, reducing blood flow and swelling.

Bloat

Bloat is always a life-threatening emergency, and veterinary intervention must always be sought as quickly as possible. Bloat makes the dog's stomach swell with gas, causing great discomfort. Severe distention of the stomach may compress the dog's heart. All breeds of dogs, but especially those with deep chests, are predisposed to bloat. Irregular feeding intervals and large meals before work or exercise increase the likelihood of bloat. Simple preventive measures include feeding small meals at frequent intervals and feeding a dog at least two hours before work or exercise. Also remember to provide your dog plenty of rest when he or she plays or works in a hot and humid environment.

Hazardous Materials and Poisonings

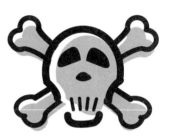

Working dogs, and in some cases your pet dog may be exposed to a great variety of hazardous materials and poisons. Dogs may ingest and inhale toxins or absorb them through their skin. If your dog has been exposed to toxins, protect the dog from further exposure and avoid exposing yourself and other people to the contaminated dog. Use protective clothing when handling the dog. If the skin has been contaminated, dogs may be washed with liberal amounts of soap (not detergent), such as a mild dishwashing soap, and water. To treat the ingestion or inhalation of toxins, veterinary advice should be sought. The National Animal Poison Control Center can also be consulted by phoning (800) 548-2423 or (900) 680-0000.

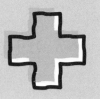

Oral and Respiratory Obstructions

Obstructions that impede swallowing or breathing make dogs gag and retch. Some dogs may also shake their heads, paw at their mouths, or cough persistently. If the problem continues or appears life-threatening, carefully—and considering your own safety—restrain the dog and see if you can identify the problem and remove the obstruction by sticking your hand down the throat. If you do not succeed, seek veterinary help promptly.

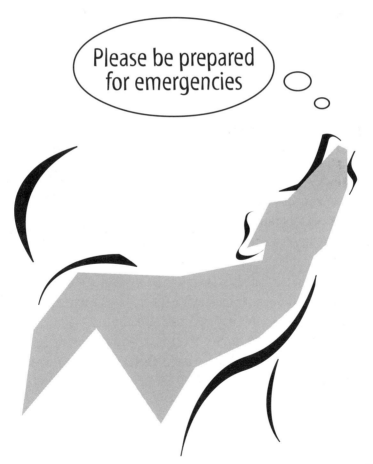

The Care of
Dogs in Disasters

The images of large-scale disasters fill our television screens and make the front pages of our newspapers on a regular basis. Typically, these reports detail cataclysmic events. We are told of earthquakes that rip through far-off provinces, leaving thousands of people homeless. We watch forest fires that rage out of control, transforming entire neighborhoods into rubble and ash. We are alerted to unusual climatic events during which once-calm streams become swollen and vicious, tearing across acres of prime farmland. Though we may never be touched by catastrophic events, disasters of a more personal nature—residential house fires, lightning strikes, automobile accidents, and illness—affect the lives of two to three million United States residents each year. Some of these less-publicized events, especially those connected with contamination or those leading to loss of power, result in evacuation or prolonged periods of isolation.

Disasters, either large or small, require you to be prepared to maintain the health and safety of you and your family *first*. For many, this will include your dogs. By taking the time to include your dogs in your disaster preparedness plans, your entire family will be able to cope better under extraordinary situations. A first step that you can take is to get in touch with the local chapter of the American Red Cross and get a copy of the Family Disaster Plan brochure (you can download a copy on the net at *www.redcross.org/disaster*). Review this brochure and use it as the basis for your disaster preparedness plan.

Several key factors need to be part of your disaster plan to ensure that your dog will have the best possible chance of survival and will be controllable during a disaster.

Planning Ahead

Preparedness is critical in reducing the impact of a disaster or preventing injury altogether. Remember that during and after a disaster, your dog will be completely dependent on you for his or her survival and well-being. The

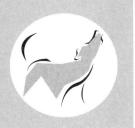

responsibility for your pet, as in your daily routine, rests solely with you. It is much better to have a plan in place prior to being faced with a disaster than to face a disaster without knowing what to do and where to go. Panic is not the answer.

Your plan must include the following key points that can be used in **EACH** situation.

1. **E**vacuation route. If you have enough time after being warned of an impending disaster, what pre-planned route will you, your family and your dogs take to escape harm?

2. **A**lternative place. If time does not permit, how will you get to a secure site on your property or the surrounding area as quickly as possible?

3. **C**ommands and training. What commands and routines must your dog know for an emergency situation?

4. **H**ealth and exercise. How fit is your dog to cope with the stress and anxiety of a disaster situation?

Your Emergency Response Plan

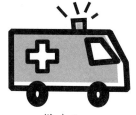

Getting ready for any disaster or emergency requires that you to take into account EACH of the above points by considering the following situations.

1. Identify the types of disasters or emergencies that are more likely to occur in your area or location. The list should be broken down into three parts: natural disasters, man-made disasters, and personal emergencies. For example, natural disasters such as tornadoes and floods are more prevalent in the Midwest, while hurricanes are more likely to occur on the East Coast.

If you live near a chemical plant or nuclear facility, you need to be prepared for the possibility of evacuation at any time. You should also consider the chances of personal disasters, such as a fire in your house or apartment complex, being involved in a car wreck, or the sudden hospitalization of the main care provider for your family or dog. Becoming aware of what your probable risks are is the first step toward developing an effective disaster plan.

2. Check your home for safety. A great number of disasters can be avoided by following some simple guidelines in the home. Be sure to have smoke detectors and, if need be, a carbon-monoxide detector installed. Check and test them regularly. Store hazardous substances in safe locations and in approved containers. Ensure that your electrical wiring and other utility lines are up to code. Have an emergency contact list near your telephones. The list should have the numbers for Poison Control, the fire and police departments, the nearest emergency room, your family doctor, and your veterinary practitioner. These precautions will save lives and might lower your homeowner's insurance premiums, too.

3. Finally, plan ahead for your dog's safety.

Training and Acclimation

A. Spend time on training your dog in basic obedience. Obedient dogs are more likely to survive an emergency and will make you more welcome guests if you are forced to evacuate and stay with your friends or leave your dog in the care of others. Several good books that provide information on how to train your dog in basic obedience are available from your local library, pet store, or bookstore. Also, many localities offer inexpensive obedience courses in association with local parks or adult education at the local schools or other community buildings. Spending some time with your

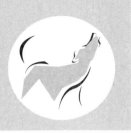

dog on obedience activities will ensure better care in an emergency situation and provide a greater degree of security in everyday situations.

B. Accustom your dog to being transported. A common reason why people fail to evacuate is because they cannot transport their dog. Buy a crate (local pet stores or national department chain stores will have several varieties) to transport your dog, or get your dog used to riding in your car by taking it on local errands and other family outings, if possible. When you bring your dog's crate home, label the crate with your dog's name, your name and address, and the name and phone number of the person with whom you will most likely be staying if you are forced to evacuate your home. It is also good to attach a note to the crate indicating if the dog has certain fears. For example, if a dog is frightened by flashlights and sirens, he will do all he can do to find the safest spot farthest away from the light or noise in which to hide. Tendencies like this should be noted.

C. Familiarize your dog with the surroundings and the people at the place you are likely to stay during an evacuation. Usually, you will stay with a family member or friend within just a few miles of your home. Bringing the dog over and letting him become acquainted under normal circumstances will lighten the stress load during an emergency. Perhaps one room will be designated as the room in which your dog will stay during and after a disaster. Take your dog to the room and allow him to explore it with you under normal circumstances. If possible, have a few of your dog's toys and a spare blanket there.

Health Issues

Disasters place many stresses on your dog, which could lead to unforeseen health problems. In order to minimize the adverse health consequences of a disaster, make sure that your dog's health is satisfactory at all times. Follow these recommendations:

29

A. Keep your dog's vaccinations current. Under disaster conditions your dog may have to mix with other dogs and animals that may be carrying diseases. Most vaccinations are repeated yearly. The rabies vaccination can be given annually or once every three years, depending on the type of vaccine used. Keep a record of the vaccination schedule to put in your disaster-preparedness kit.

B. Exercise your dog regularly. By walking your dog several times a week, your pet will maintain a healthy body weight. Disasters place extraordinary physical stresses on dogs. Keeping your dog in shape will prepare him for these rigors.

C. Make sure your dog has a permanent form of identification. The most economical solution is to have your pet wear a collar and tags. However, you can now have your dog identified with a microchip or tattoo.

D. If your dog is on a prescription, special medications, or a special diet, keep a list of the names of these items handy or ask your veterinarian for a written copy of your dog's medications and ailments. Dogs being treated for cancer, eye, or skin conditions, for example, may need a multitude of drugs every day that have long names that can easily be forgotten. After a disaster, veterinary care may not be available from your regular veterinarian. Therefore, if your dog needs treatment, you will need a copy of your dog's records to ensure proper care without interruption.

The Emergency Response Plan

1. IF YOU HAVE TO EVACUATE, ALWAYS TAKE YOUR DOG(S) WITH YOU.

2. Decide on primary and secondary places where you and your family will meet if you have to leave your home. These locations should be within a mile or two of your home.

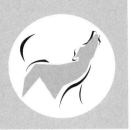

3. Decide on a person outside of your area/state through whom members of your family can relay information. Often you cannot phone into a disaster area, but it is possible to phone out. Your primary outside contact will be the conduit for all family members to relay information about other family members. You can also relay information on the care of your dog through your out-of-area phone contact.

4. Let friends and family know where you will be staying with your dog if you are evacuated.

5. Make sure you know the official evacuation routes in your home area.

6. If you think you may not be able to care for your dog in a disaster, decide who will be able to provide that care. For example, make arrangements for dog care with neighbors, family, or friends. Make sure they have keys to your house and leave information on your current location, how you can be reached, and instructions for your dog.

7. The best emergency plans involve many people and systems that provide help for each other. Encourage a number of people and groups to get involved, including family, friends, and neighbors. You should also ask local veterinarians and dog-breed and owners' clubs to get involved. An effective and proven method of ensuring mutual help in a disaster is to establish a telephone tree. Telephone trees work when one person phones two friends to see if they need help or to request help. These two people phone another two, and so on. Soon many people know who needs help and what help can be provided.

8. Write down your plans and practice them. You should practice evacuating until you are sure you can evacuate your family and your dogs within a few minutes.

Prepare a Disaster Kit

You should prepare a disaster kit for each dog in your care. Kits and their contents should be easily retrieved and kept in rodent- and ant-proof containers. Do not store kits in the kitchen or garage because house fires start in these areas 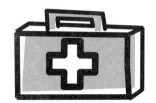 most frequently. Remember to check the contents of your disaster kits twice a year when you change to or from daylight savings time. Be sure to rotate all stored foods every two months. What should your disaster kit contain?

1. Include collars with tags, harnesses, and leashes for each dog. Owners frequently complain of the lack of leashes after disasters. Not having a leash means you may not be able to walk your dog and others may not feel safe around you and your dog.

2. Pack a muzzle or materials to make a muzzle (see page 6). Even the most gentle animal may become aggressive when frightened, and disasters are frightening.

3. Keep an extra store of your dog's regular food. A diet change may lead to stomach upsets, especially under the stressful conditions of disasters.

4. Pack toys and blankets with which your dog is familiar.

5. Include a supply of bottled drinking water. Dogs normally consume water at a rate of one quart for each ten pounds of body weight per day.

6. Have bowls for food and water for each dog you own.

7. Pack paper towels, plastic bags, and spray disinfectant for easy and sanitary cleanup of your dog's waste.

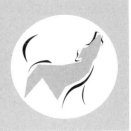

8. Include a recent photo of your dog.

9. Pack a manual can opener.

10. Include quarters for use in public telephones.

11. If your dog requires regular medication, keep a current copy of your dog's prescription or extra supplies of its medication in your disaster-preparedness kit. Consult your veterinarian on this issue for his or her advice. Make sure to keep a listing so that you will know when to replace expired medications.

12. Make copies of your dog's vaccination, health, and ownership records and place them in your dog's disaster-preparedness kit. You might need to board your dogs. Boarding kennels will need these records.

13. Include some basic first-aid materials (see page 49). Useful items for a first-aid kit would include materials to treat minor wounds, to remove small foreign bodies, and to stop excessive bleeding.

When Disaster Strikes

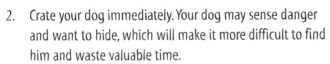

1. Stay calm and assess the situation. By following the above guidelines, you will be prepared for what is about to happen.

2. Crate your dog immediately. Your dog may sense danger and want to hide, which will make it more difficult to find him and waste valuable time.

3. Be aware of your dog's temperament. In the commotion of a disaster, your dog may become anxious and could react by biting.

4. Listen to the Emergency Alert System (EAS) on your battery-operated radio for latest evacuation instructions. Be sure to listen for special arrangements for people with dogs. Follow official recommendations when you make evacuation decisions. (You might browse the EAS Web site — *http://www.eas.net* — at your convenience prior to a disaster to see what services are available.)

5. Never put yourself or others at risk. Do not attempt to rescue your dog if your life or health or that of others may be placed in danger.

Being Separated from Your Dog

Some situations – for example, a disaster is declared while you are at work or you may fall ill or be injured at work – will make it nearly impossible to evacuate your dog. Also, shelters may not be set up to deal with pets due to local public-health regulations. In rare circumstances, owners have had to leave their dogs behind as a last resort.

If you must leave your dog behind, follow these guidelines:

1. Choose a room in your house that can be easily cleaned, has few electrical outlets, and can be closed off. Bathrooms are an especially good choice.

2. Keep your dogs separated from other pets you need to leave behind.

3. Do not tie your dogs to posts, fences, trees, or other objects. Confining your dog in this way might lead to its death by drowning, burning, or being struck by heavy objects.

4. Do not let your dogs loose. Roaming dogs are a public health threat and are your responsibility in case they cause injury or other damage. During and after many disasters, animal control officers have no choice but to treat roaming dogs as strays. Once captured, the dogs are either put up for adoption or euthanized.

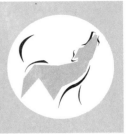

5. If possible, make arrangements with neighbors, family, or friends to care for your dog. Let them know in which room your dog is staying and how they can get in contact with you.

6. Do not leave unfamiliar foods and treats for your dog. He or she may overeat, which could lead to intestinal problems. Provide water in a heavy bowl that can't be tipped over. Be careful to close the lid on your toilet since the water supply might become contaminated.

7. Attach labels (that you prepared earlier) in a visible spot so that rescue workers will know that dogs are in the home. The labels should indicate how many dogs are in the home, the dogs' names, where they are, and where you can be contacted.

8. Post commands with which your dog is familiar, preferably in a location near the room where the dogs are staying.

9. If you've lost your dog, pay daily visits to local humane shelters, animal control facilities, veterinary offices, and kennels. A phone call is often not as effective as a personal visit. You can also post photos of your dog in several high-traffic areas. If your dog has a tattoo, microchip, or other permanent identification, your chances of finding your dog will be much greater. Collars and tags can easily be lost during a disaster.

Recovering from a Disaster

When a disaster has passed, it is not uncommon to find that once-familiar surroundings have been altered, sometimes severely. Since dogs rely on visual and olfactory (scent) clues to find their way around, they can become very disoriented. The following guidelines will help you and your dog through the recovery period:

1. When bringing your dog into new surroundings, do not let it out of its crate until it is calm. Bring the crate to a closed-off room before opening the crate's door. Let your dog feel free to come out when it feels safe.

2. You should check your dog for any signs of injury or possible exposure to chemicals or other hazardous substances. If you are concerned about your dog's health, contact your veterinarian before you attempt to treat the problem.

3. Listen to the radio for instructions from Emergency Management personnel as to whether the environment is safe for you and your dog. Be careful when you let your dog out for the first few times. Familiar landmarks and scents may be gone. You should also be aware of other dangers, such as unleashed pets, bad water, storm debris, and downed power lines.

4. If your dog has been without food or water for more than a day, offer your dog only small amounts of food and water several times throughout the next few days. You should increase the volume to a normal amount during a two-to-four-day period. Do not let your dog drink tap water unless it has been declared safe for humans to drink, too.

5. Let your dog have plenty of uninterrupted sleep. If you still have your dog's favorite toys, encourage him or her to play. This will help to promote recovery from the stress and trauma of the disaster.

6. Avoid unfamiliar activities with your dog, such as bathing, excessive exercise, or using dietary supplements. Try to avoid diet changes and irregular feeding schedules. Do not allow your dog to swim in or drink from floodwaters.

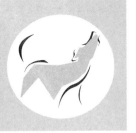

7. Share your experiences with friends and family. Encourage your children to describe their experiences. Talking about your experiences will help you deal with them and offers stress relief. If any of your family members experiences extreme stress, consider seeking professional counseling. Recovery from the stresses of a disaster is often faster when guided by experienced professionals.

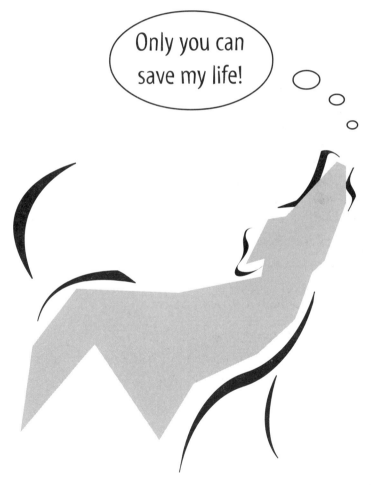

Specialty Help for Your Dog

The veterinary profession is organized in many ways similar to the human medical profession, with general practitioners and specialty practices. Most of the time your dog's health can be maintained by regular visits to your veterinarian, who is probably a general practitioner. However, if your dog has an unusual problem, your veterinarian will refer you to a veterinary specialist. The following contact addresses summarize which specialties may be of interest to you as a dog owner and may help you in selecting a specialist.

General Veterinary Practitioners

Contacts for your state's Veterinary Medical Association can be obtained from telephone directories (usually in the state capital) or from the American Veterinary Medical Association.

General Questions on Veterinary Care

American Veterinary Medical Association
1931 North Meacham Road, Ste. 100
Schaumburg, IL 60173-4360
800.248.2862

American Animal Hospital Association
PO Box 150899
Denver, CO 80215-0899
303.986.2800

Specialty Veterinary Disciplines

Many states have schools or colleges of veterinary medicine at a university. These usually employ a variety of veterinary specialists.

Behavioral Problems

American College of Veterinary Behaviorists
College of Veterinary Medicine
University of Georgia
Athens, GA 30602
706.542.8343

Skin Problems

American College of Veterinary Dermatology
2122 Worthingwoods Blvd.
Powell, OH 43065
614.292.7105

Emergency Medical Care

American College of Veterinary Emergency and Critical Care
School of Veterinary Medicine
Tufts University
200 Westboro Road
North Grafton, MA 01536
508.839.7950

Veterinary Emergency and Critical Care Society
Auburn University
Dept. of Small Animal Medicine
Auburn, AL 36849
334.844.4690

American College of Veterinary Internal Medicine
7175 West Jefferson Ave., Ste. 2125
Lakewood, CO 80235-2320
303.980.7136

Nutritional and Dietary Consultations

American College of Veterinary Nutrition
College of Veterinary Medicine
Dept. of Small Animal Medicine and Surgery
Texas A & M University
College Station, TX 77843-4474

Eye Problems

American College of Veterinary Ophthalmologists
Dept. of Veterinary Clinical Sciences
Louisiana State University
Baton Rouge, LA 70803
504.346.3333

Specialty Surgical Procedures

American College of Veterinary Surgeons
4340 East West Highway, #401
Bethesda, MD 20814-4411
301.718.6504

Teeth Problems

American Veterinary Dental College
Dept. of Surgical and Radiological Sciences
School of Veterinary Medicine
Davis, CA 95616
916.754.8254

Poisoning

National Animal Poison Control Center
University of Illinois
College of Veterinary Medicine
2001 South Lincoln
Urbana, IL 61801
900.680.0000 (24-hour hotline for fee)
800.548.2423 (consultations for fee)

Canine and Breed Associations

American Boarding Kennels Association
4575 Galley Road, Ste. 400A
Colorado Springs, CO 80913
719.591.1113

American Kennel Club
51 Madison Avenue
New York, NY 10010
212.696.8200

Information on the Care of Animals in Disasters

Animals in Disasters, Independent Study Courses (free)
Module A (15-010): Awareness and Preparedness
Module B (15-011): Community Planning
Federal Emergency Management Agency
EMI - Independent Study Program
16825 South Seton Avenue
Emmitsburg, MD 21727-9986

American Humane Association
63 Inverness Drive East
Englewood, CO 80112-5117
303.792.9900

Humane Society of the United States
2100 L Street, NW
Washington, DC 20037
202.452.1100

United Animals Nation
2233 Benton Street
Santa Clara, CA 95050
408.984.6702

American Academy on Veterinary Disaster Medicine
3910 Morehouse Road
West Lafayette, IN 47906-5409
765.463.4493

American Red Cross
Attn: Public Inquiry Office
6th floor
8111 Gatehouse Road
Falls Church, VA 22042
(or contact your local American Red Cross office)

Checklist

Check off the items you have prepared.

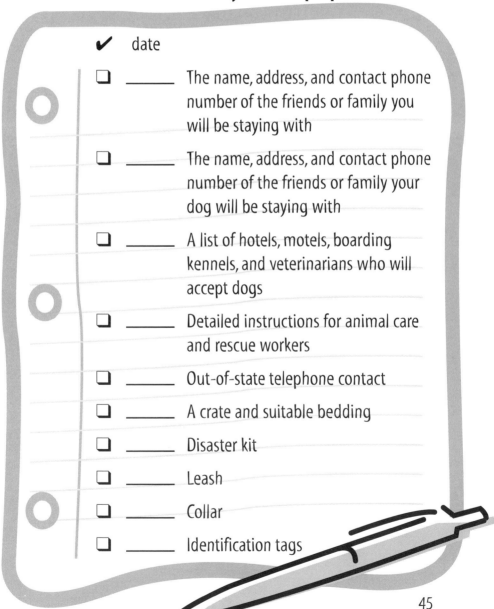

✔ date

❏ _____ The name, address, and contact phone number of the friends or family you will be staying with

❏ _____ The name, address, and contact phone number of the friends or family your dog will be staying with

❏ _____ A list of hotels, motels, boarding kennels, and veterinarians who will accept dogs

❏ _____ Detailed instructions for animal care and rescue workers

❏ _____ Out-of-state telephone contact

❏ _____ A crate and suitable bedding

❏ _____ Disaster kit

❏ _____ Leash

❏ _____ Collar

❏ _____ Identification tags

✔ date

❑ _____ Muzzle

❑ _____ Food

❑ _____ Water

❑ _____ Plastic bags, paper towels, and newspapers for waste disposal

❑ _____ Copies of current medical and vaccination records

❑ _____ Copies of health certificates

❑ _____ Copies of prescriptions

❑ _____ Current photos

❑ _____ Zip lock bags

❑ _____ First aid kit (see page 49)

❑ _____ Quarters (25¢)

❑ _____ Battery operated radio

Your Dog's Vital Signs

If you are not familiar with how to gather this information, we recommend that you consult your veterinarian. The many breeds and sizes of dogs also mean that there is a large range of normal values for dogs. Therefore, collecting and interpreting the normal vital signs of your dog should be demonstrated by a professional. The following information is useful:

_____

Name (common, registered)

_____

Breed

_____

Description (breed colors, distinguishing marks)

_____   _____

Age   Normal adult weight

_____   _____

Normal resting heart rate   Normal resting respiration rate

_____   _____

Normal body temperature   Normal capillary refill time

Your Dog's Vital Signs cont'd

Hydration status

Normal demeanor

Regular diet (brand, amount, how often fed)

Regular exercise schedule

Regular veterinarian

First Aid Kit Checklist

**You should only include material that
you know how to use properly and safely.**

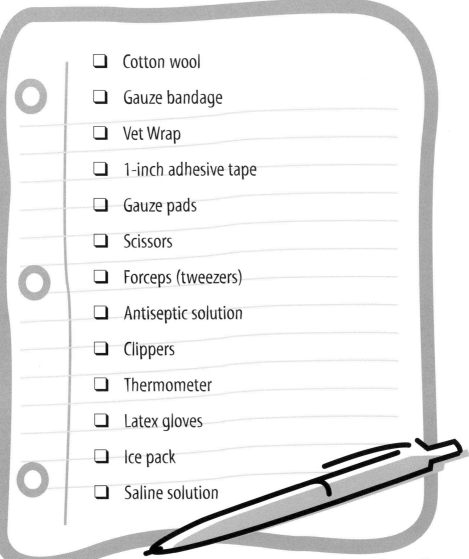

- ❏ Cotton wool
- ❏ Gauze bandage
- ❏ Vet Wrap
- ❏ 1-inch adhesive tape
- ❏ Gauze pads
- ❏ Scissors
- ❏ Forceps (tweezers)
- ❏ Antiseptic solution
- ❏ Clippers
- ❏ Thermometer
- ❏ Latex gloves
- ❏ Ice pack
- ❏ Saline solution

Commands that Your Dog Recognizes

Describe spoken instructions and the hand and body motions you use for the following commands.

To make my dog sit.

Spoken instruction	Hand and body motions

To make my dog remain where it is.

Spoken instruction	Hand and body motions

To make my dog lie down.

Spoken instruction	Hand and body motions

To make my dog come to me.

Spoken instruction	Hand and body motions

To make my dog stop doing an activity.

Spoken instruction	Hand and body motions

Rover Asks for Your Help

Money donated to the National Association of Search and Rescue contributes to research and service programs that enhance the care of animals in disasters and to locate lost and trapped victims.

Name _____

Address _____

City _____

State _____ Zip Code _____

Enclosed is a donation for the following amount (please check):

❑ $10   ❑ $100

❑ $50   ❑ other _____

Send all donations to:

National Association of Search and Rescue
4500 Southgate Place, Suite 100
Chantilly, VA 20151-1714
Telephone: (703) 222-6277
FAX: (703) 222-6283
Email Information: info@nasar.org
http://www.nasar.org/

and specify that your donation is to support NASAR programs that are active in disasters.

Books of Related Interest

Between Pets and People
The Importance of Animal Companionship

by Alan Beck and Aaron Katcher
foreword by Elizabeth Marshall Thomas

This revised edition, with additional data, case studies, and an expanded reference section—including Internet resources— analyzes the surprisingly complex relationships we have with our pets. This book emphasizes an important lesson— we should accept ourselves and others in the uncrucial way that pets accept us and come to terms with our own animal nature.

"Their interpretations may startle readers.... Clearly, humans need companion animals, and this book tells us why."
— Publishers Weekly

1996
336 Pages
ISBN 1-55753-077-7

Published by
Purdue University Press

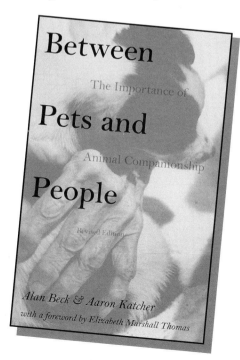

Books of Related Interest

Veterinary Medical School Admission Requirements in the United States and Canada

compiled by the Association of American Veterinary Medical Colleges

This compact volume, which is updated annually, gives a general overview of the application process, including detailed information on the Veterinary Medical Colleges Application Service and residency requirements. Each of the thirty-one veterinary medical schools in the United States and Canada provides information about campuses, deadlines, specific prerequisites, expenses, and special programs. Extensive tables provide data on veterinary medical applications and acceptances over the last nineteen years.

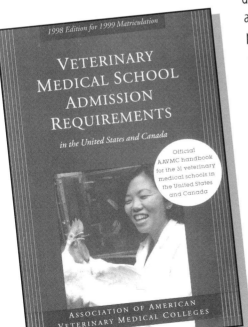

1998 Edition for 1999 Matriculation
184 Pages
ISBN 1-55753-132-3

Published by
Purdue University Press